LIGHT VISION

LIGHT VISION

MOHAMAD   J.   VAJED

Quotations of poems by Hafiz were taken with permission from the book "The Gift:
poems by Hafiz the Great Sufi Master", translations by Daniel Ladinsky, published by the Penguin
Putnam Inc. 375 Hudson Street, New York, N.Y. 10014, USA. Copyright Daniel Ladinsky, 1999

Printed in the United States of America

10   9   8   7   6   5   4   3   2   1

ISBN 0-9666915-1-2

Library of Congress Control Number 00-131405

LC Control Number

00 131405

Originally Published by *Graphic Ways Publishing* in 2000
Reissued by REGENT PRESS in 2009
ISBN 13: 978-1-58790-167-6
ISBN 10: 1-587890-167-6
Library of Congress Control # 2009924888
www.regentpress.net   regentpress@mindspring.com

For Diane,
the light of my life

God is the light of heavens and earth

KORAN 24:35

And God Said, "Let there be light"; and there was light

GENESIS 1:3

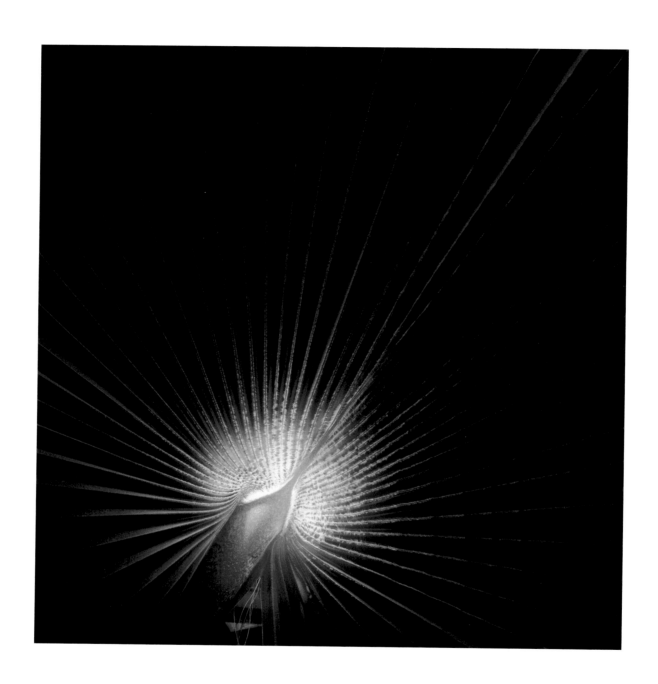

PREFACE

"There is nothing new under the heavens" says the Bible, and this book is no exception. Most of the pictures are of ordinary subjects that have been photographed many times before. The differences exist only in the way they were perceived and are presented here.

A general rule in photography, as in other forms of art, is "know yourself and be yourself." We all influence each other. Some influence by established photographers is inevitable and beneficial, so long as it does not manifest itself as mere imitation and duplication. The work of others serves best as a guide to improvement and refinement of technical abilities.

Ideally, the creative process develops its wings deep in the cocoon of our individuality. Photographers strive to develop a unique style, and their work may become recognizable, even without a signature. I have tried to achieve that, but the degree of my success is not for me to judge.

Significant achievement in any endeavor cannot be realized without the aid and guidance of others. I am indebted to and wish to acknowledge the following individuals: Ansel Adams for his unfailing passion and his advancement of the art of photography (I was fortunate to attend a few of his lectures). His books have been very helpful; especially those with information concerning the zone system; Morley Baer (page 61), Henry Gilpin and John Sexton for their valuable and informative workshops; John Wimberley, who started it all for me and graciously wrote the introduction to this book; and my dear friends and colleagues Abdorreza Saidian, M.D. and Stephen Petuyan, M.D., whose constant encouragement was invaluable to me and the continuation of my work. My special thanks also to many others who in some way have helped me to bring this book to completion.

This preface would be incomplete without mentioning my personal views regarding photography. For me, it liberates the soul. When I am taking a picture, I feel as if I am sharing in the creative power of the Almighty.

Photography literally means writing with light, which is the source of all being. Without it there would be no life, and no photography. It is ironic that we see everything with light, yet without things we cannot perceive light. My real quest in photography is light itself; I use form to carry light, as a cup carries wine. My earnest desire is to know light so intimately that ultimately I become a part of it. The object of all our struggles is union with the Infinite, which is the Light. The contemporary Iranian poetess Forugh Farrokhzad (1934-1966) eloquently put it this way:

نهایت تمامی نیروها پیوستن است، پیوستن

به اصل روشن خورشید

و ریختن به شعور نور

The end of all forces is union

union

with the luminous source

of the sun

and

pouring

into the consciousness of light.

(translated by Zahra Taheri Haghighy, Ph.D)

Mohamad J. Vajed

INTRODUCTION

It is said that a poet is born, not made. If that is true, then it is certain that Mohamad J. Vajed was born a poet. He entered this world in the beautiful southern Iranian city of Shiraz which, for many centuries, has been known as the Persian "City of Roses and Wine." It was in Shiraz that Persia's two greatest poets, Sa'di and Hafiz, flowered. Both Sa'di (Sheikh Muslihu'd-dīn Sa'di, c. 1200-1290), and Hafiz (Shams-ud-dīn Muhammad, c. 1320-1389), wrote in the Persian ecstatic mystical tradition of their longing for God and of their experience of God in everyday life. More recently, Mohamad's father, Mohamad Ja'far, also a renowned poet, continued that tradition, passing it on to his son, who was raised in an atmosphere of ancient and modern art and spirituality. In a way similar to the role of opera in Italy, poetry is the national art of Persia. This rich milieu had a profound effect on Mohamad.

As a child, Mohamad found that he had a deep connection with the natural world: "I had a very intimate relationship with nature, and it's still in me." Thus, it was only natural that Mohamad would become a poet / photographer of nature, seeing in the natural world the hand of its creator, and the reflection of his own soul: "I love nature. When I go outside, my soul is happy." Spiritual joy is apparent in his photographs, whether as the radiant explosion of a "Palm Leaf", or in the profound intimacy which radiates warmly from "Portrait of a Young Woman."

Mohamad trained as a physician, and even there, art was present: "Medicine is an art; you cure the patient, not the disease." He credits the practice of medicine with helping him develop his keen faculty of seeing, of noticing: "Observation is the first thing in medicine." This is the noticing not only of details, but also the overall patterns which the details form or suggest. Seeing in this manner is, of course, the basis of photographic seeing, and, if the photographer is fortunate enough to have the soul of a poet, as does Mohamad, the camera records not only the light of the outer world, but also the inner light of the photographer. As Minor White wrote: "In light the inner and the outer stand mirrored."

After seeing an exhibition of my photographs in 1979, Mohamad took up the camera. He realized that he had found a medium with which to record his own poetry of light: "I saw the power and beauty of black and white; I just fell in love." Photography, as time allowed, became a passion and gave form to Mohamad's love of nature: "From childhood I could see what others ignored. I saw in every speck that beauty is everywhere." It is light that makes seeing possible, and light is not only outer illumination, it is the prime characteristic and symbol of consciousness, that luminosity within us which perceives, and is, light.

Like a great starving beast

My body is quivering

Fixed

On the scent

Of

Light.

— *Hafiz*

With the momentous discovery in the 1840's of light-sensitive materials on which an image could be "fixed", artists finally had a medium which recorded light directly. Previously, light could only be written or sung about, painted or drawn. The definition of light as "something that makes things visible" was and is the physical basis of photography. Film, like Hafiz's "great starving beast", exists for its encounter with light. This "outer light" is the factor which fulfills the destiny of the film. Film is not concerned with the intensity of light, as long as it receives a sufficient dose, nor does it worry about the nature or meaning of the image formed within its emulsion. Photography, at its most elemental, simply records light, any light. At this level, photography is a superb transcriber of visual descriptions, an impeccable memory without a soul or spiritual context. It is only the poet with a camera who can, in moments of deepest clarity and passion, reveal, rather than merely record, the world. Just as the film surrenders itself to its destiny, the poet/photographer gives all of himself to the moment of making a picture. Much like a camera lens, he simply and clearly focuses his inner light of consciousness into the moment. When this happens, the resulting picture is a double image, composed of two sources of light, outer and inner, which are, paradoxically, one.

> A poet is someone
> Who can pour light into a cup
> Then raise it to nourish
> Your beautiful parched, holy mouth.
>
> —*Hafiz*

According to virtually all esoteric and religious insight, consciousness is indeed light, and the source of that light is infinite. To practice photography as a poet is to knowingly or unknowingly tred a spiritual path, and the history of photography is replete with references, both clear and veiled, to this fact. From Alfred Stieglitz—who could assert, "To show the moment to itself is to liberate the moment." To Edward Weston, who wrote, "Clouds, torsos, shells, peppers, trees, rocks, smokestacks are but interdependent, interrelated parts of a whole, which is life"—photographers have discovered or been drawn to the spiritual.

The influence of one's inner light on seeing is to enable the direct perception of wholeness in the world, not only that of separate objects and events. This way of perceiving is essential to art. Everything in a finished work, regardless of the medium, must be in relationship, in other words, form a whole. The individual character of that relationship is an expression of wholeness through the photographer, not only in using the camera, but in facilitating (and getting out of the way of) his own inner light. Both inner technique and outer technique are equal facets of one's development as a photographer. The spiritual hunger that is the foundation of the sustained effort to develop both simultaneously, and to bring them into productive relationship, is a hallmark of the poet with a camera. As Hafiz wrote:

You need to become a pen
In the Sun's hand

We need for the earth to sing
Through our pores and eyes.

The body will again become restless
Until your soul paints all its beauty
Upon the sky.

Don't tell me, dear ones,
That what Hafiz says is not true,

For when the heart tastes of its glorious destiny
And you awake to our constant need
For your love

God's lute will beg
For your
Hands.

Human consciousness has, as one of its valued characteristics, the perception of light. Reflected or radiant light is focused by the lens of the eye onto the retina, the immediate instrument of external vision. From there, electro-chemical impulses convey information through the optic nerve to the brain. In some unknown way, visual imagery is formed within the brain, which is then perceived *as if* it were outside ourselves and composed of the light which originally entered the eye.

The mechanism is similar to that of cable television. There, a retina-like detector in the TV camera is stimulated by light, from which a signal is generated and transmitted through a cable to the television. The signal is then converted back into light by the television's picture tube. But, just as that light is not the original light of the TV studio, the light we see by in daily life is not that to which the eye responded. Thus, even when externally stimulated, all the light which we perceive is actually produced internally and is composed of the same luminance present in dreams and visions.

Inwardly, light entices us like moths, and our hunger for its ultimate source is a yearning for spiritual enlightenment. It is insight, or *inner-sight,* which recognizes the essential unity of that which appears to be outer and inner perceptions of light. That which we perceive as outside is actually within us, and that which we perceive as our inner world, our inner light, is in truth the universe.

> At times of insight
> the illumination of surfaces
> reveals I AM within.
> — *Minor White*

Mohamad says of the times when he is photographing: "I am so focused that if a train came, I wouldn't see or hear it." Concentration of all of one's attention is, of course, a form of meditation. As this meditation is practiced day by day, more of oneself can be brought into the present moment and focused on the object of one's photographic attention. Eventually all of oneself may become focused, and, at that moment, inner wholeness is achieved, and unity with the "outside" world is experienced. The result is beautifully expressed by Mohamad: "Whatever I see guides me to the real light."

In images of plants and flowers, portraits, and studies of industrial forms, Mohamad is able to bring about the marriage of inner and outer light. The rich and ancient Persian tradition that he embodies transmutes every line of his pictures into something as sublimely beautiful as Arabic calligraphy. Here, Mohamad reveals himself to be "a pen in the Sun's hand."

A tradition lives as long as each generation provides those individuals who give it form. Mohamad, inheriting the poetic / mystical tradition of his father, and nurtured by the cultural bounty of Shiraz, has successfully evolved the heart of Persian poetry into photography. It is Mohamad of whom I am reminded when I read *The Vintage Man* by Hafiz:

The

Difference

Between a good artist

And a great one

Is:

The novice

Will often lay down his tool

Or brush

Then pick up an invisible club
On the mind's table

And helplessly smash the easels and
Jade.

Whereas the vintage man
No longer hurts himself or anyone

And keeps on
Sculpting

Light.

John Wimberley
Palo Alto, California

LIGHT VISION

Different Arrangement #1 *1981*

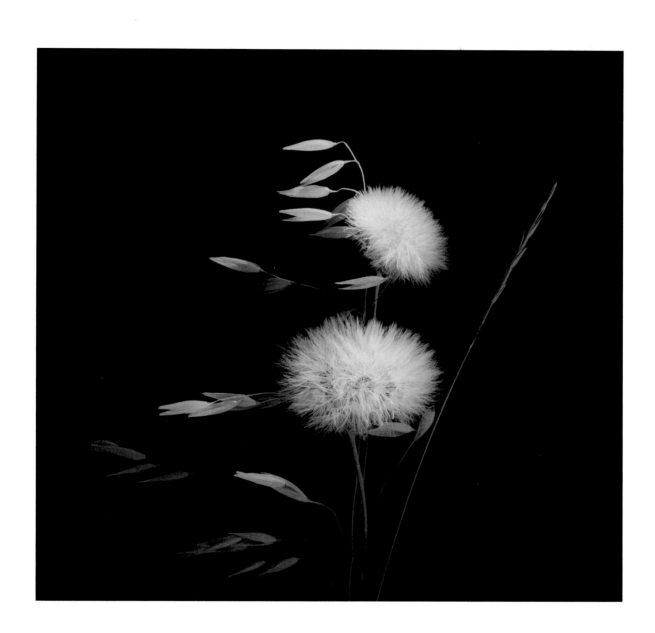

Calla Lily *1995*

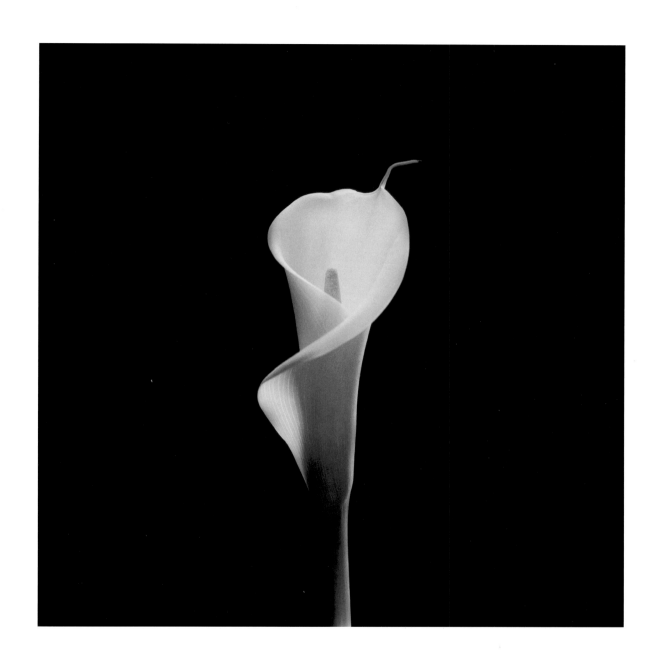

Portrait of a Young Woman *1978*

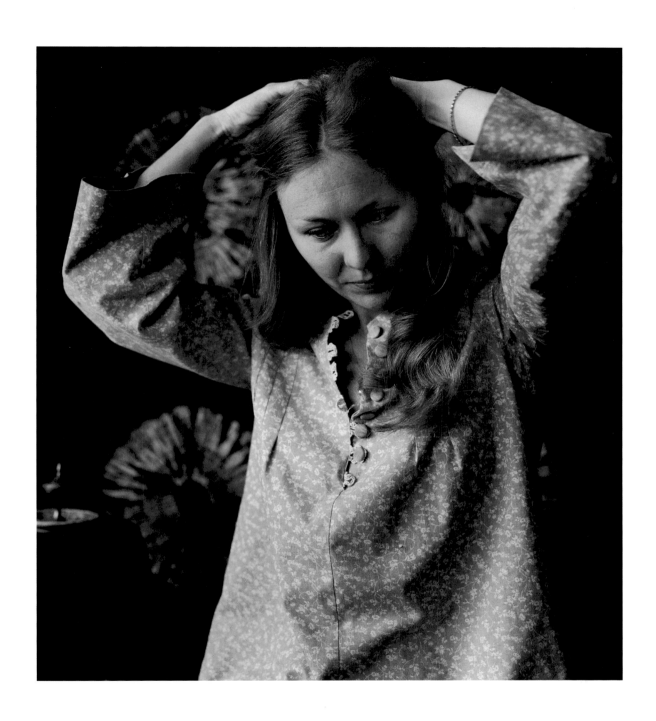

Magnolia *1989*

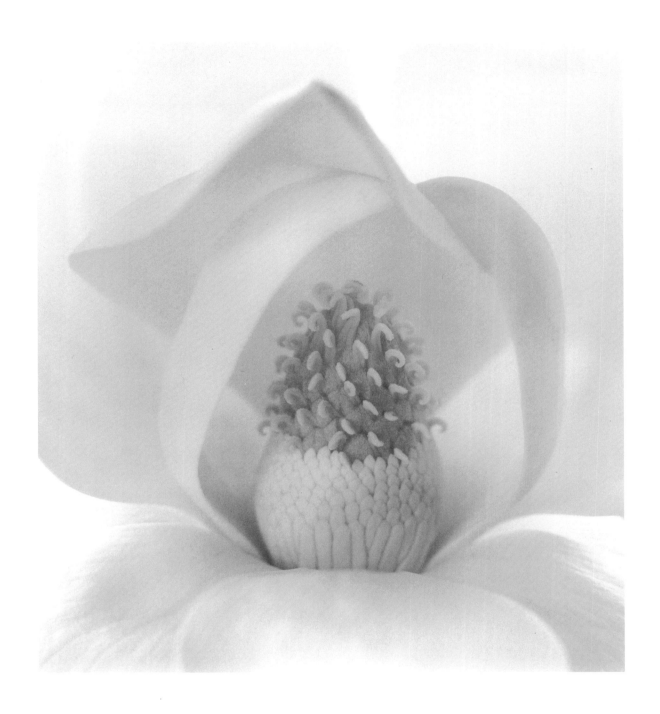

Sunflower *1997*

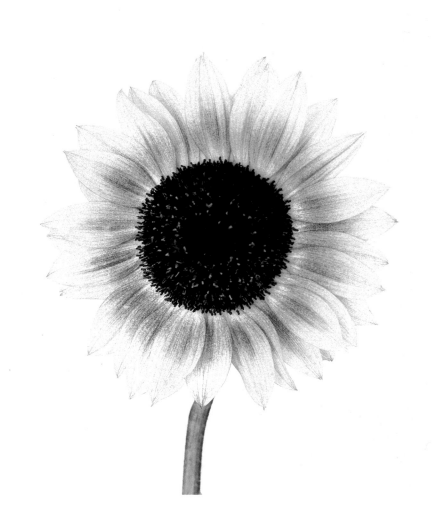

Storage Tank, Kauai *1989*

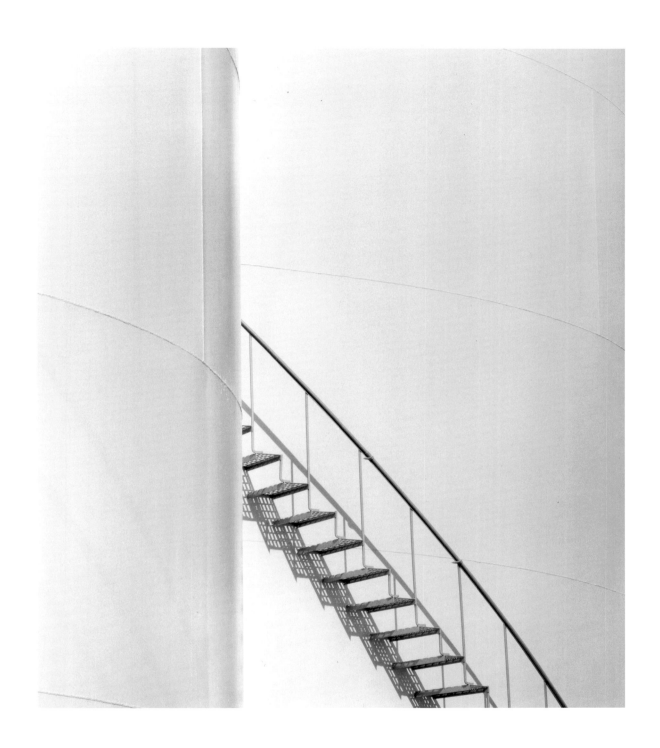

Different Arrangement #2 *1981*

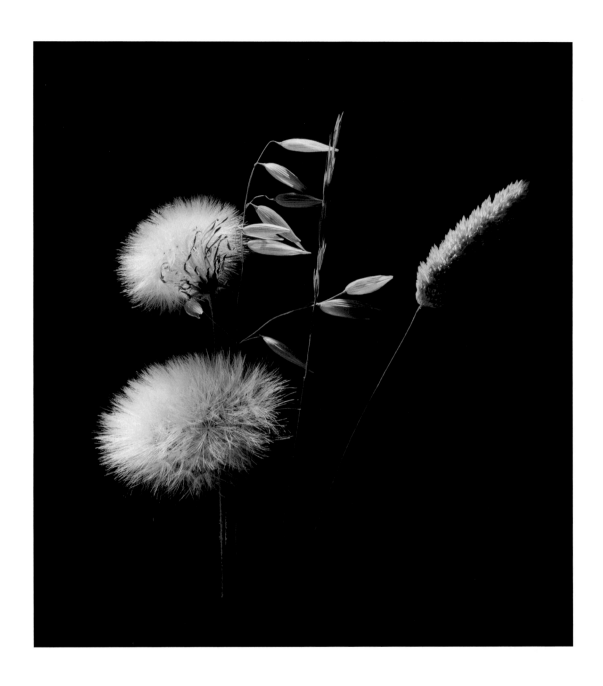

Closeup, sunflower *1997*

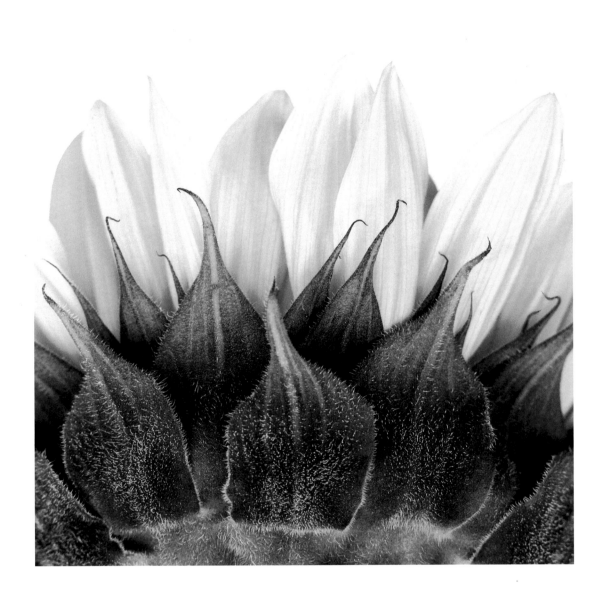

Stones, Tree, and Mist *1986*

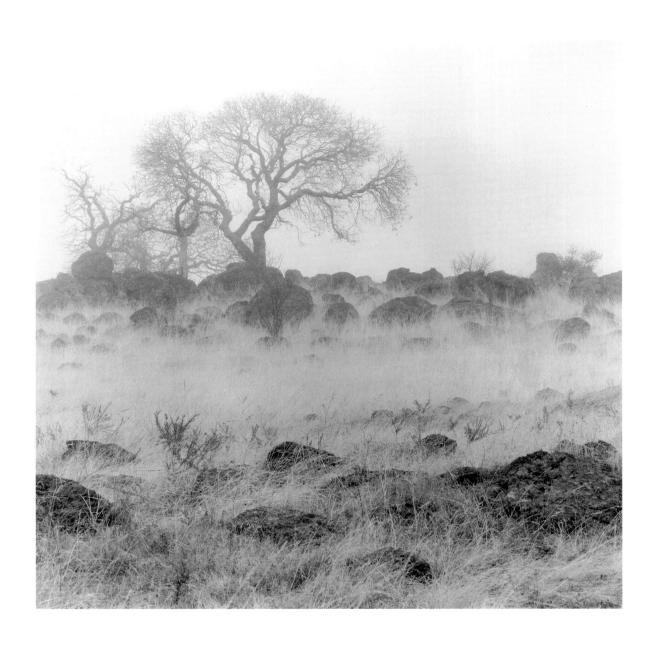

Portrait of an Old Man *1990*

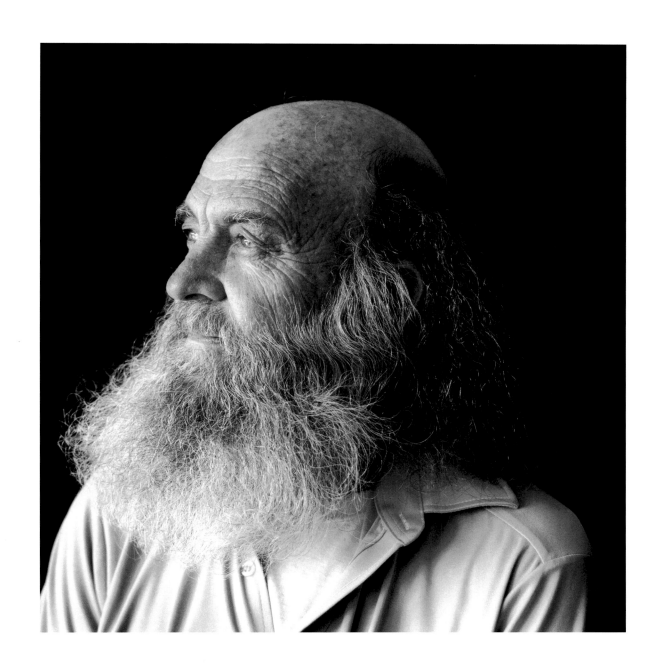

Jerusalem Artichoke Flower *1997*

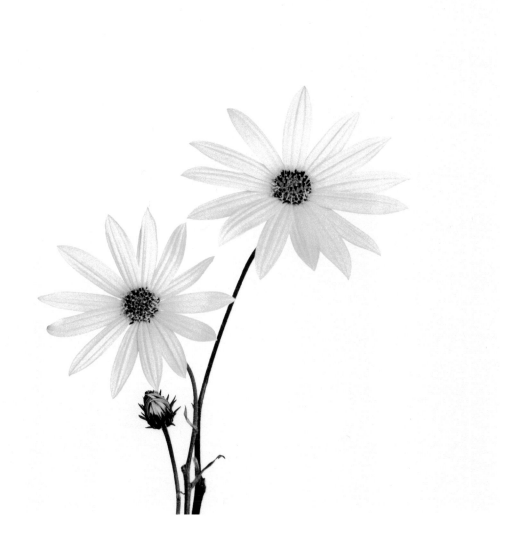

Metamorphosis *1999*

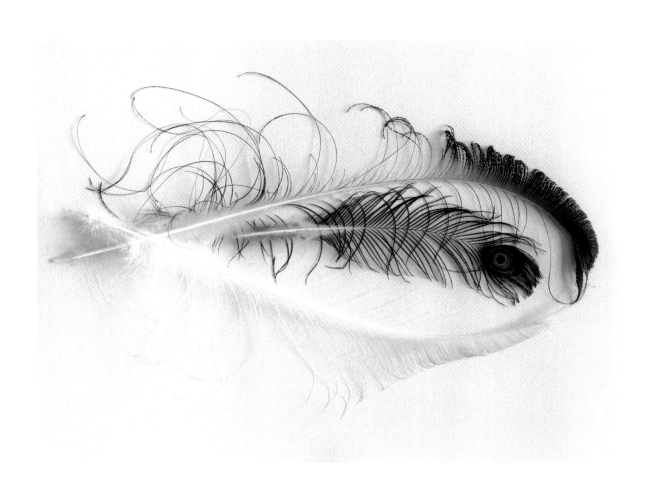

Palm Leaves, Hawaii *1991*

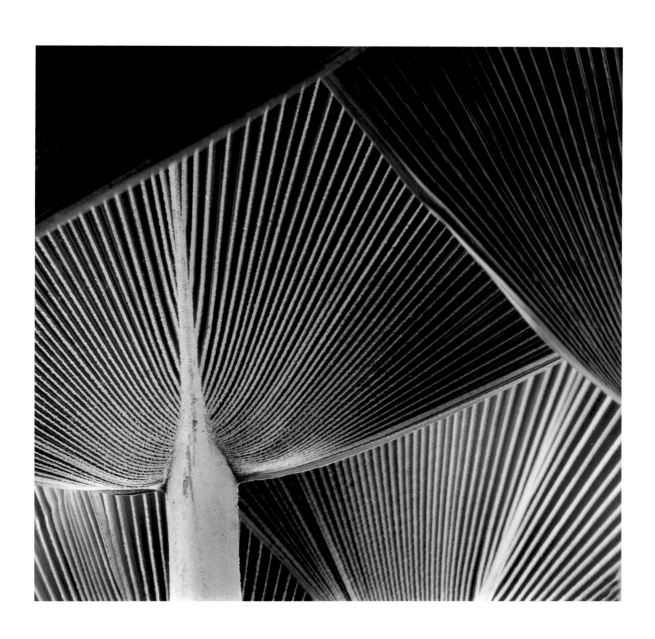

Orchard in fog *1998*

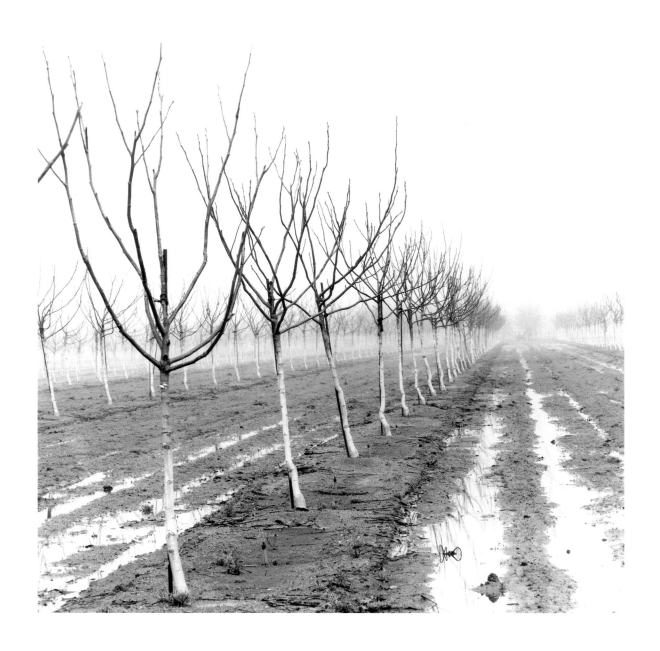

Shell *1996*

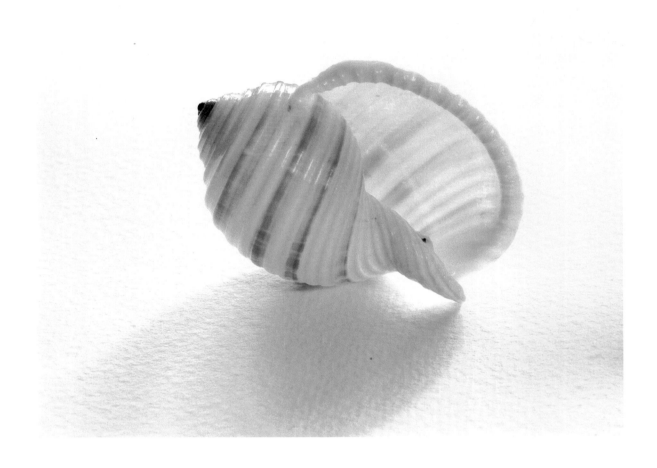

Hemlock, Green Gulch *1992*

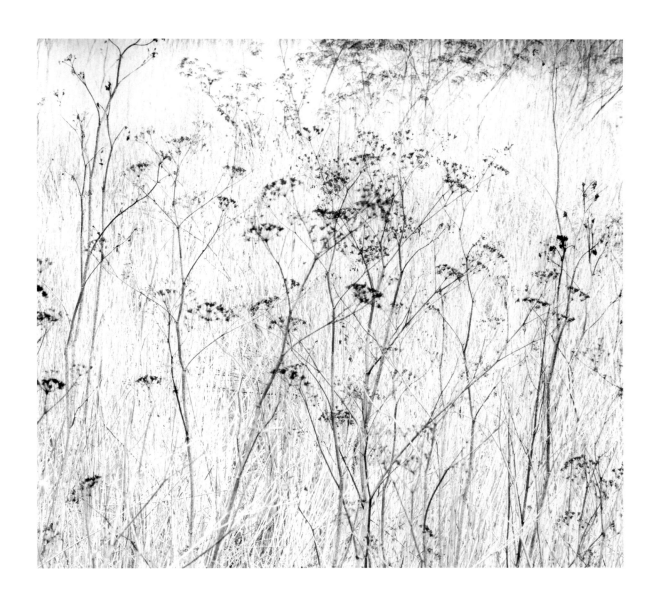

Sandstone, Point Lobos *1996*

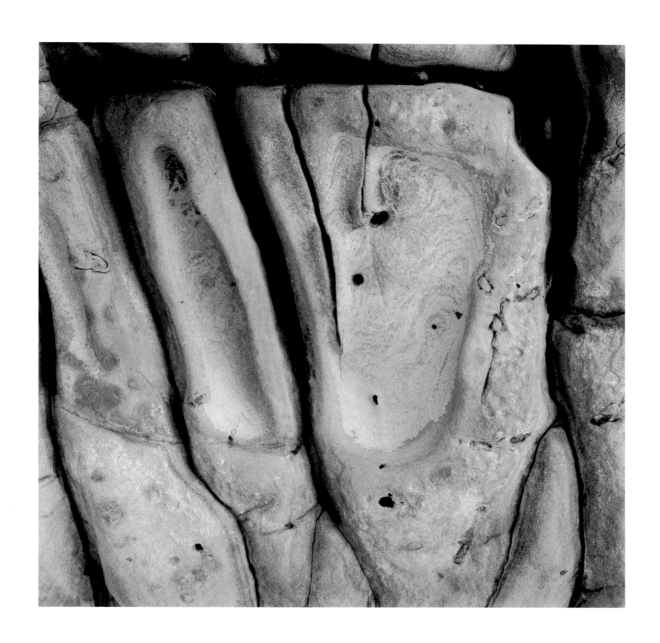

Lava & Driftwood *1995*

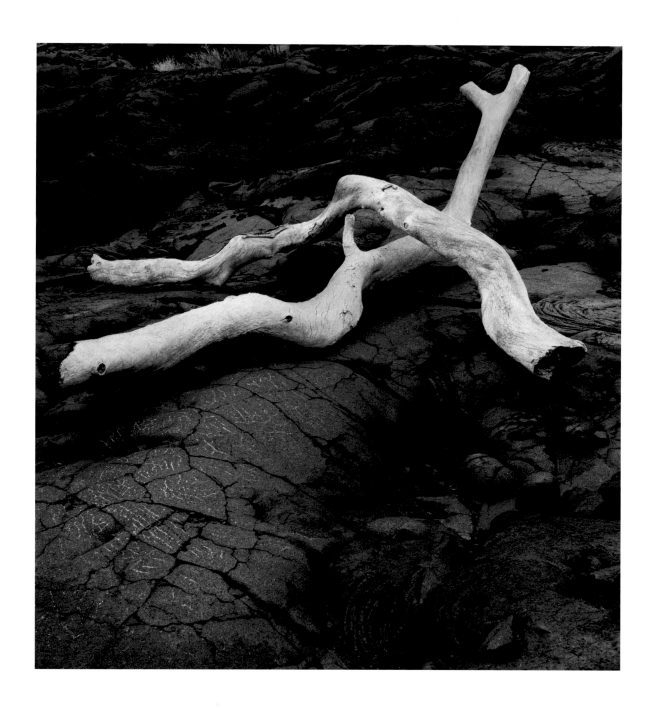

Yosemite in Winter *1990*

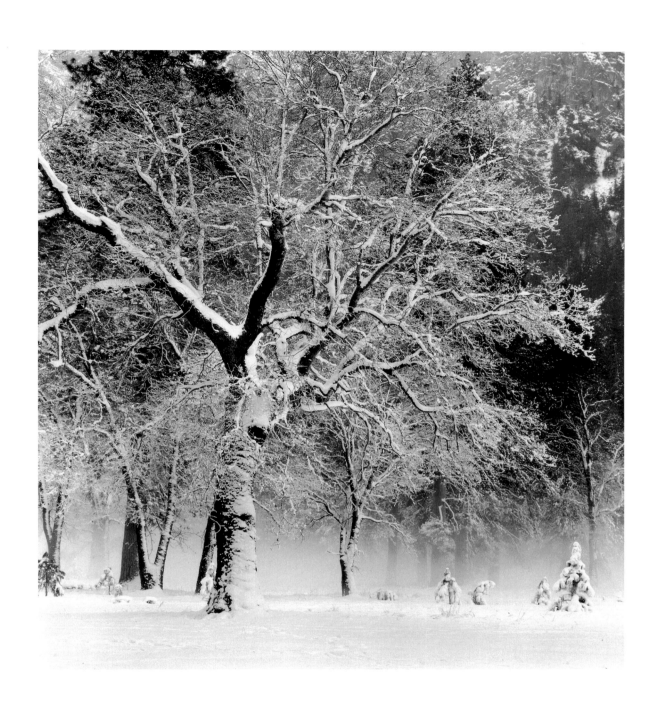

Cactus and Moon *1985*

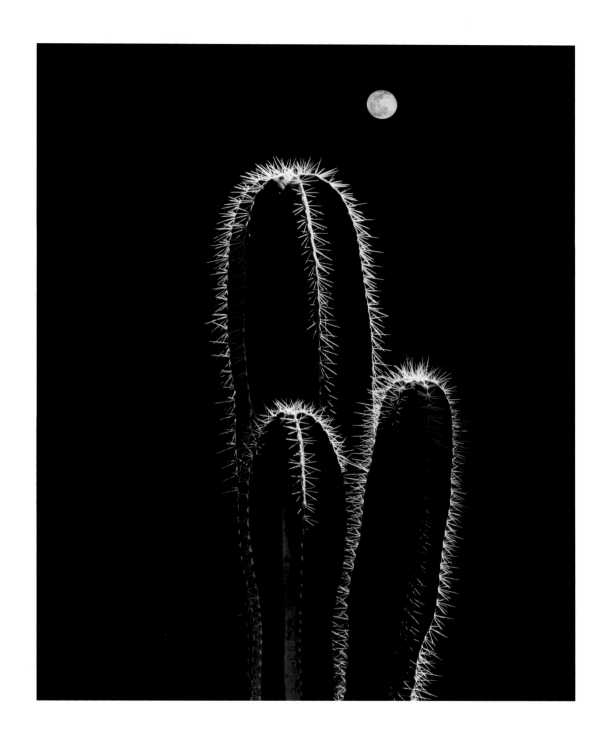

Morley Baer *1991*

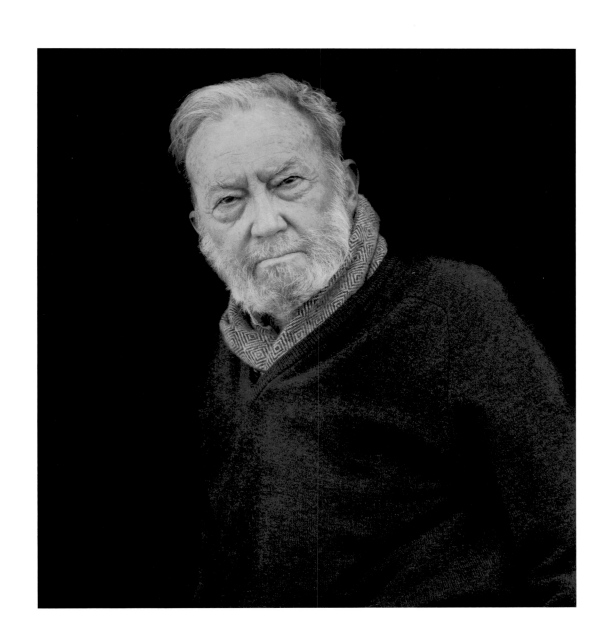

Silver Dollar Shadow *1987*

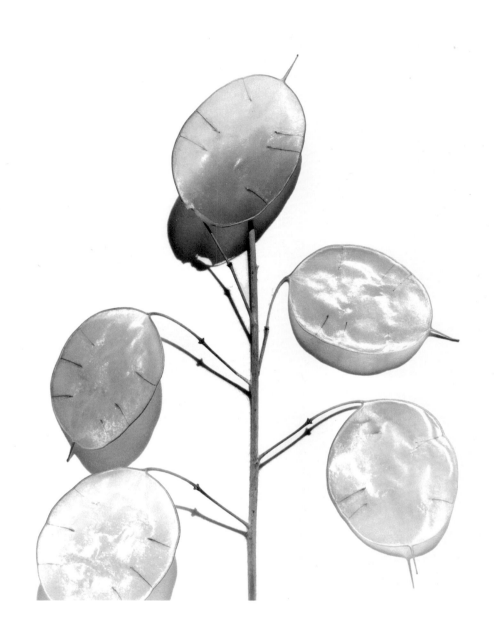

Single Leaf *1989*

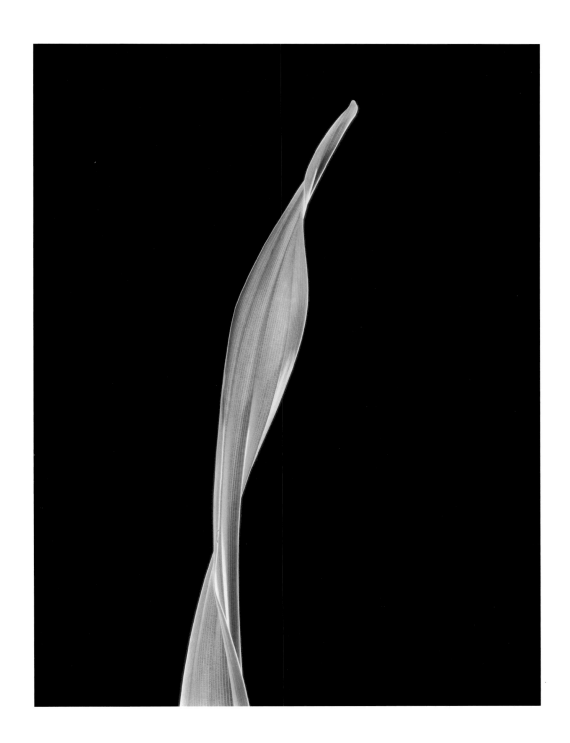

Storage Tank, Hawaii *1995*

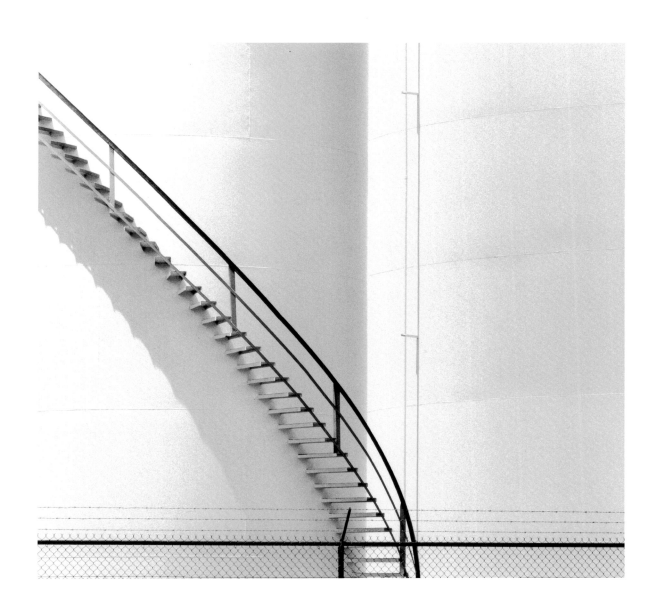

Chambered Nautilus *1986*

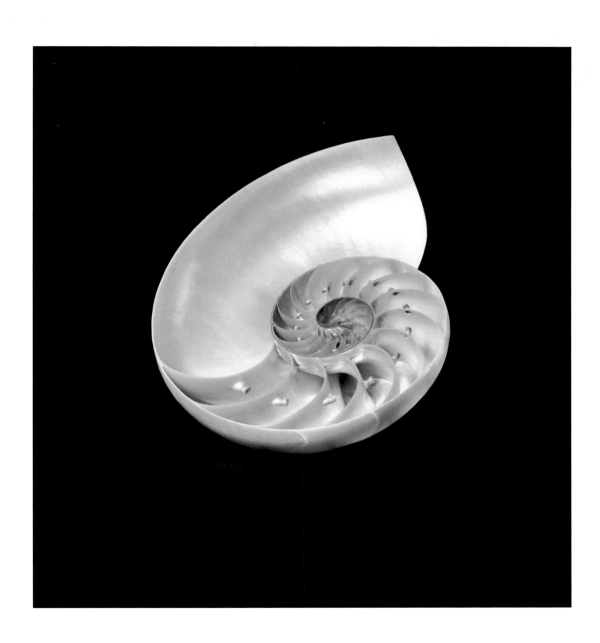

Old Brewery Tanks, San Francisco *1983*

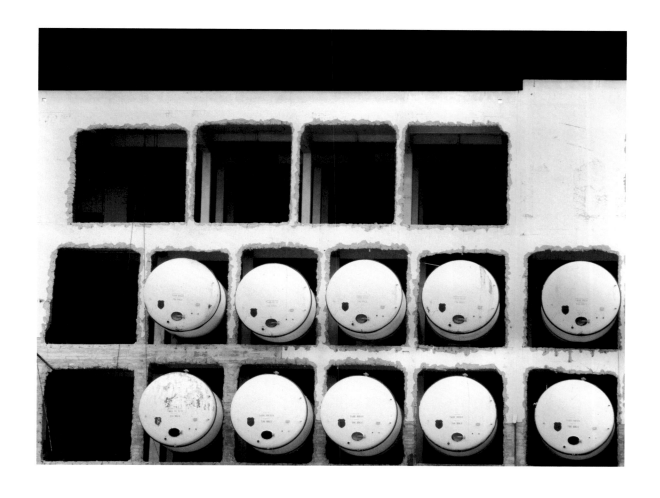

Stems, Wheat *1991*

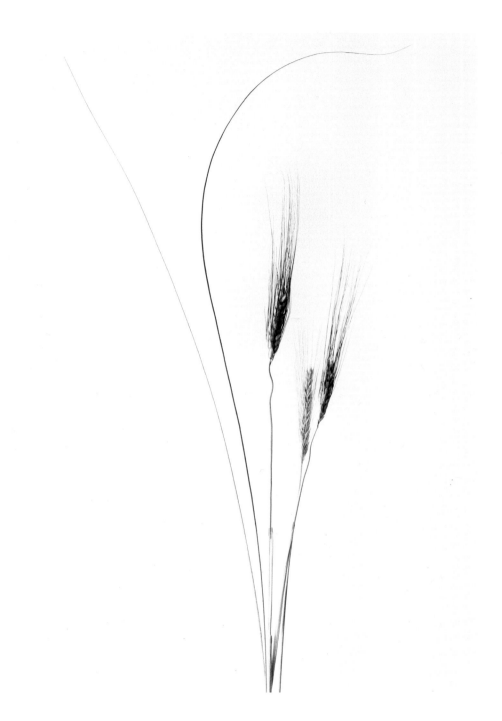

Reflection, Pond #1 *1989*

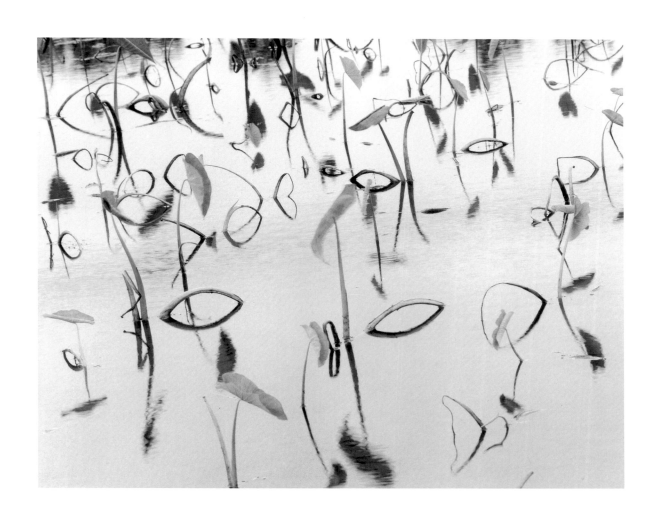

Reflection, Pond #2 *1989*

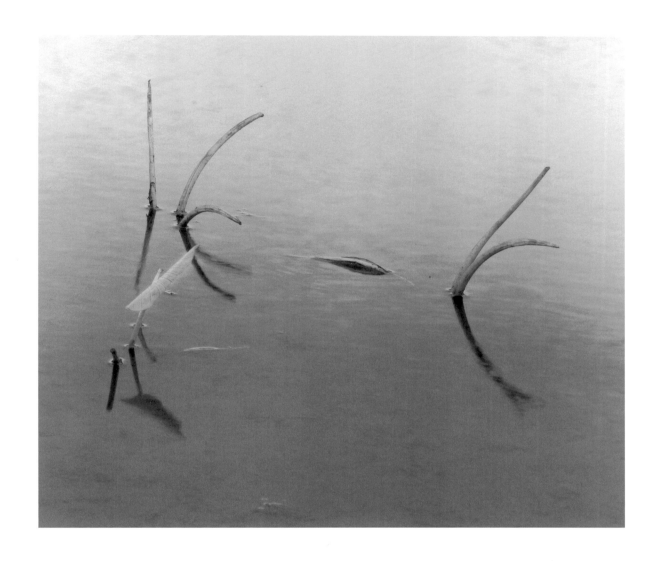

Eggshells *1991*

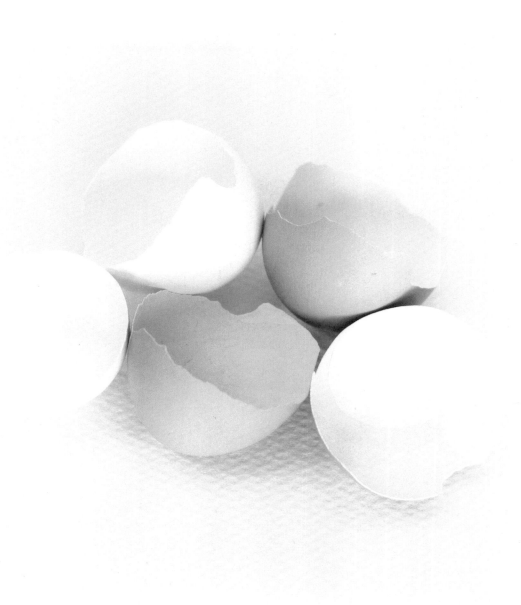

Plumeria *1991*

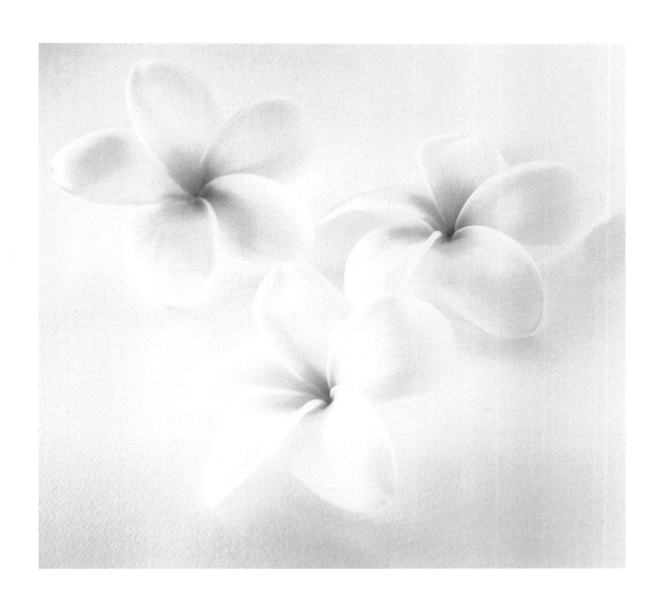

Crystal Springs Reservoir *1988*

Storage Tank *1998*

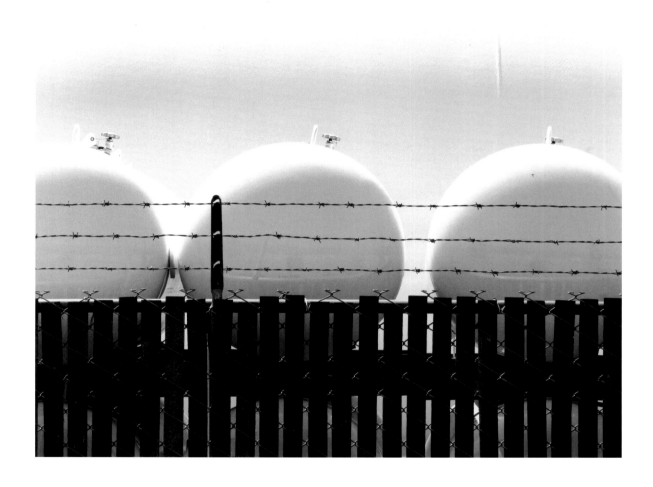

Protea *1995*

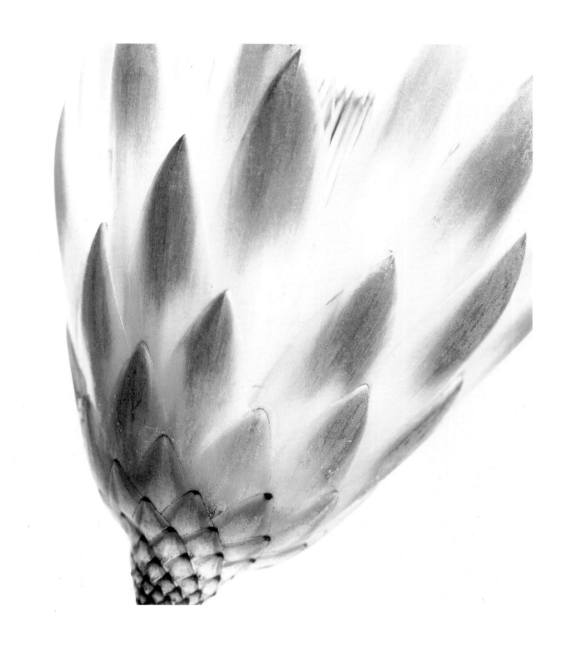

Cosmos *1996*

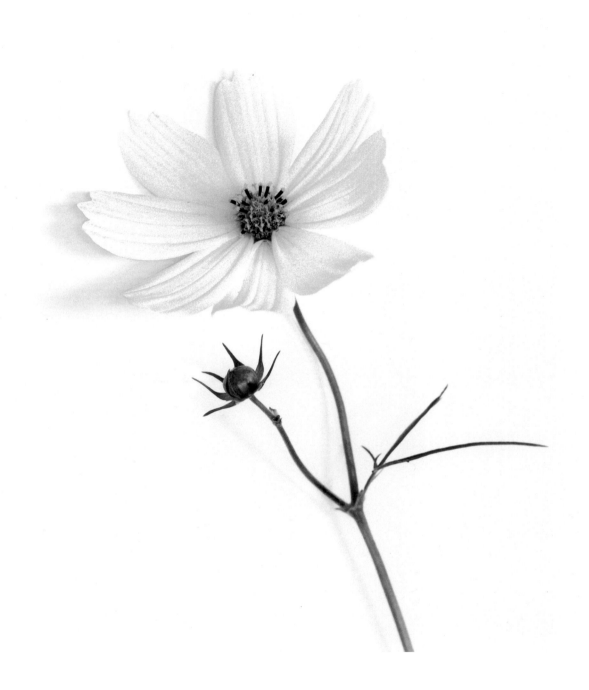

Meadow, Green Gulch *1991*

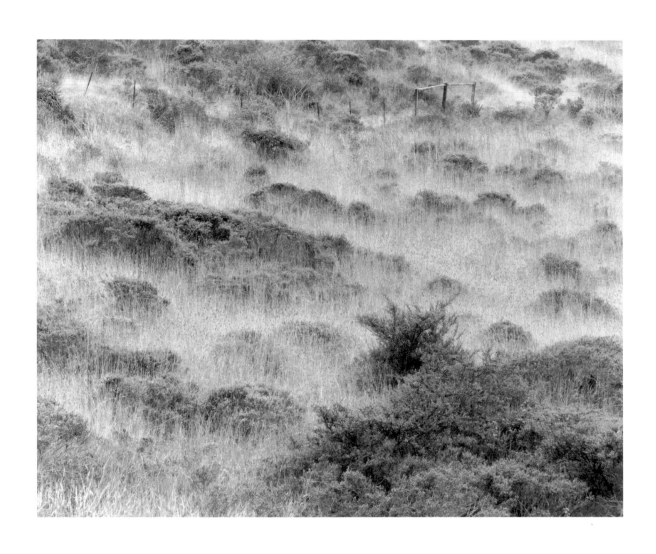

Orchid *1997*

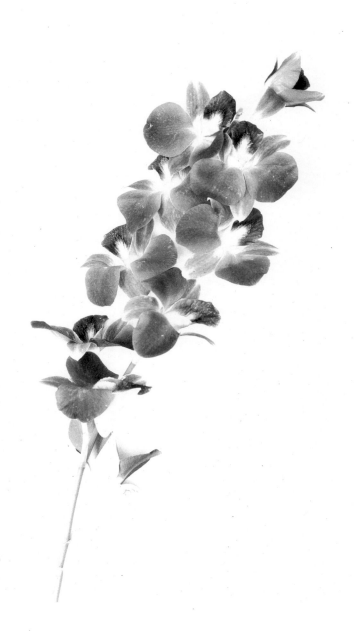

Merced River, Yosemite National Park *1996*

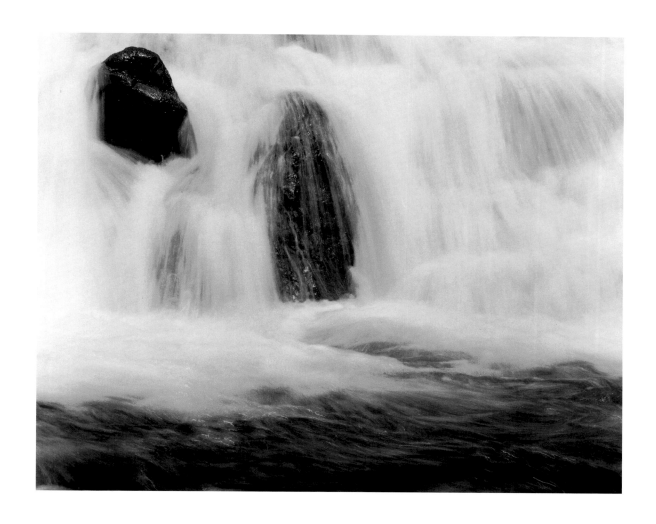

Pear *1997*

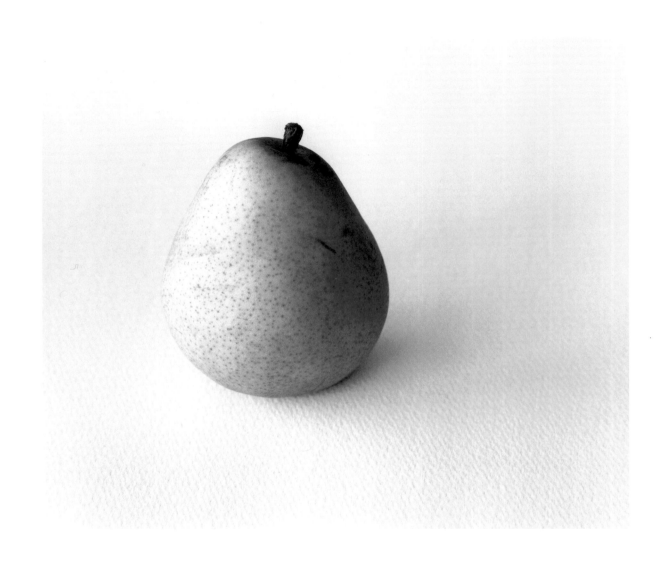

Foxglove *1990*

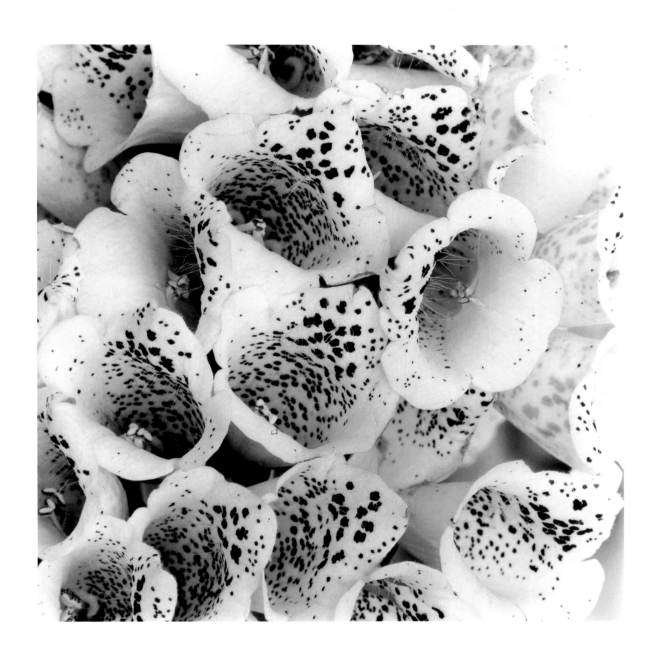

Asian Apple *1994*

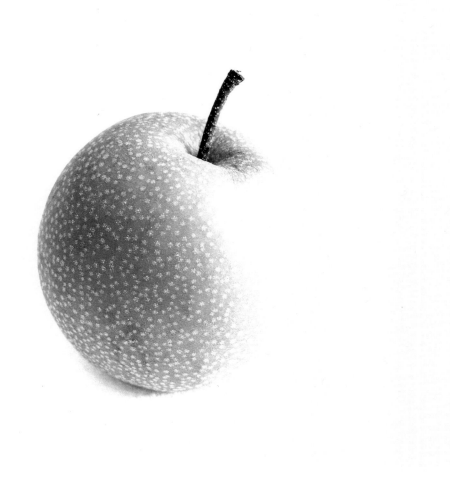

Feather *1995*

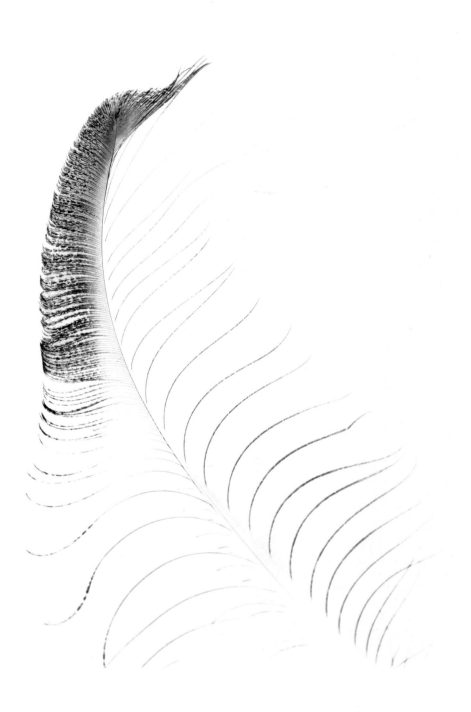

Phaleonopsis *1994*

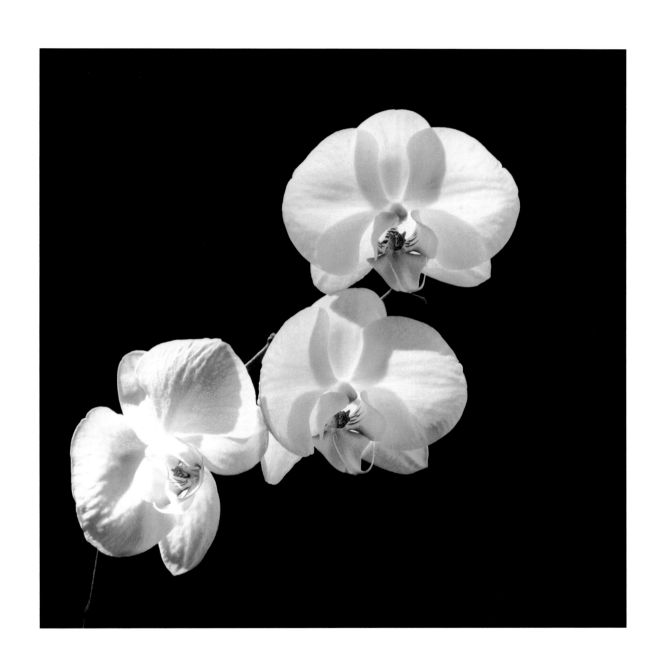

Gladiola *1989*

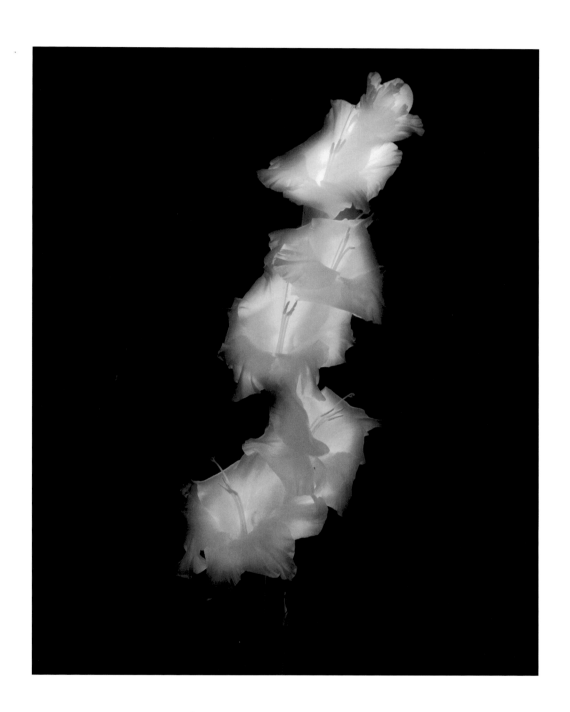

Starburst *1990*

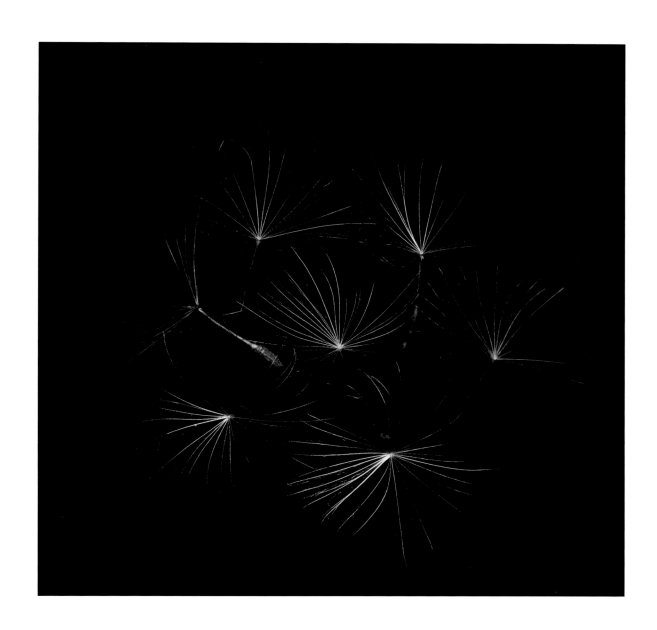

TECHNICAL NOTES

All the photographs in this book were taken with the 6 x 6 cm medium format Hasselblad 500 C/M camera. I used the 150 mm and 250 mm Sonnar lenses with professional shade attached, (always on a sturdy Tiltall tripod). For close up work, 21 and 55 extension tubes were utilized. In the early years I used Ilford FP4 film and Pyro-Metol developer (WD2D) with excellent results. However, due to the known toxicity of Pyrogallol, I later switched to Kodak HC110 (dilution B) and Agfa Pan APX 100 film with El 50. Most images in this book were taken at f/16−f/22 and 1/2−1 second. Fiber based graded papers of different brands, including Agfa Insignia, Forte Elegance Bromoform, and Oriental Seagull were used and toned in Selenium for archival preservation.

Printed by Gardner Lithography
Buena Park, California

The photographs were reproduced in the laser Fultone® process
and printed on 60 lb. Centura Gloss Cover

Bound by Roswell Bookbinding
Phoenix, Arizona